UPDOG

DEADLY DISEASES

COVID-19

The Coronavirus Disease

Jackie Golusky

Lerner Publications ◆ Minneapolis

Lerner Publications Company
An imprint of Lerner Publishing Group, Inc.
241 First Avenue North
Minneapolis, MN 55401 USA

For reading levels and more information, look up this title at www.lernerbooks.com.

Main body text set in ITC Franklin Gothic Std.
Typeface provided by Adobe Systems.

Designer: Mary Ross

Library of Congress Cataloging-in-Publication Data

Names: Golusky, Jackie, 1996– author.
Title: COVID-19 : the coronavirus disease / Jackie Golusky.
Description: Minneapolis : Lerner Publications , [2022] | Series: Deadly diseases (UpDog Books) | Includes bibliographical references and index. | Audience: Ages 8–11 | Audience: Grades 2–3 | Summary: "Scientists and health-care workers around the world are battling COVID-19. Find out how the disease attacks the human body and see how people are fighting back"— Provided by publisher.
Identifiers: LCCN 2020043816 (print) | LCCN 2020043817 (ebook) | ISBN 9781728428345 (library binding) | ISBN 9781728431239 (paperback) | ISBN 9781728430614 (ebook)
Subjects: LCSH: COVID-19 (Disease)—Juvenile literature.
Classification: LCC RA644.C67 G65 2022 (print) | LCC RA644.C67 (ebook) | DDC 614.5/92414—dc23

LC record available at https://lccn.loc.gov/2020043816
LC ebook record available at https://lccn.loc.gov/2020043817

Manufactured in the United States of America
1-49371-49475-1/21/2021

Table of Contents

A New Disease

In 2020, COVID-19 shocked the world.

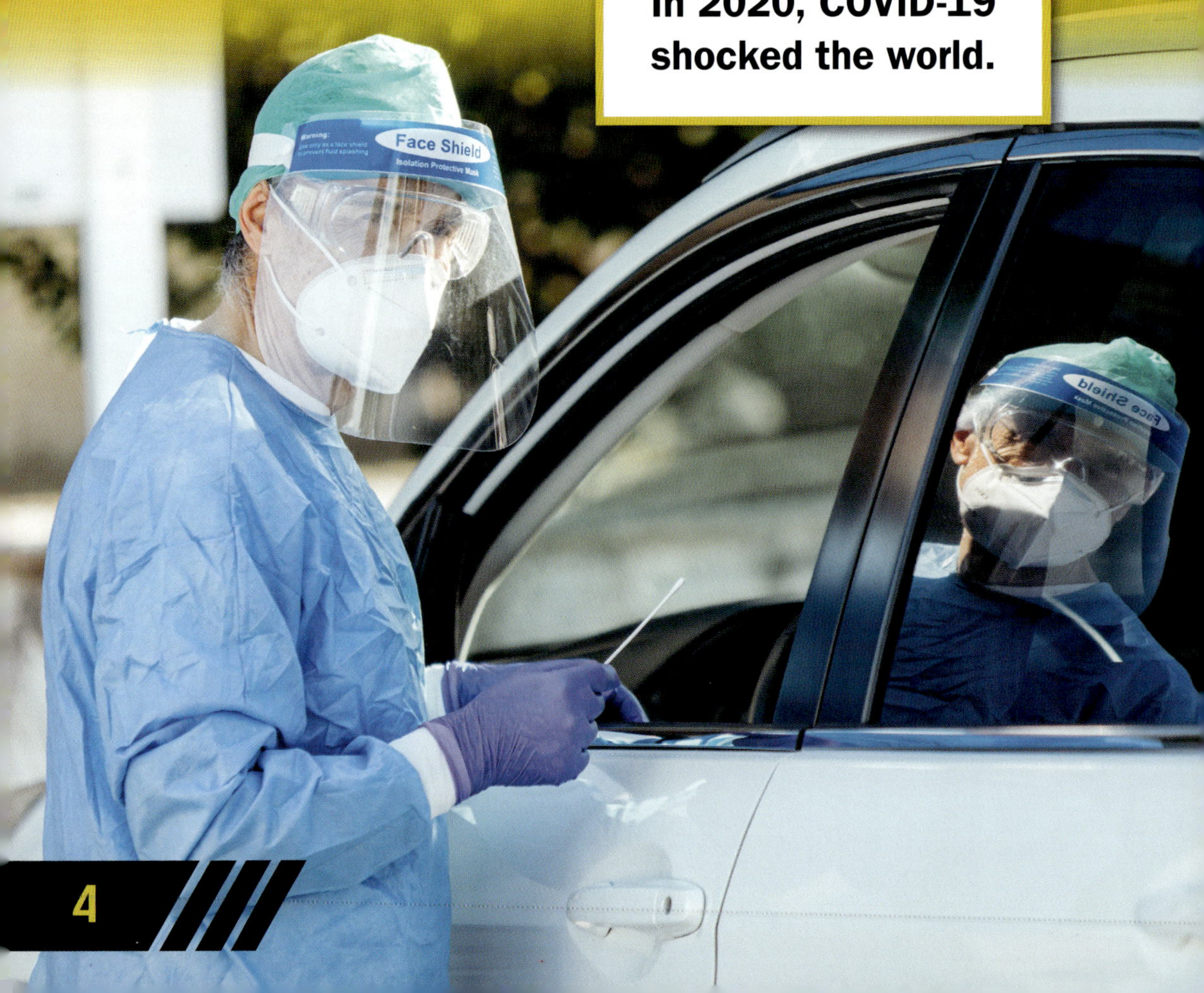

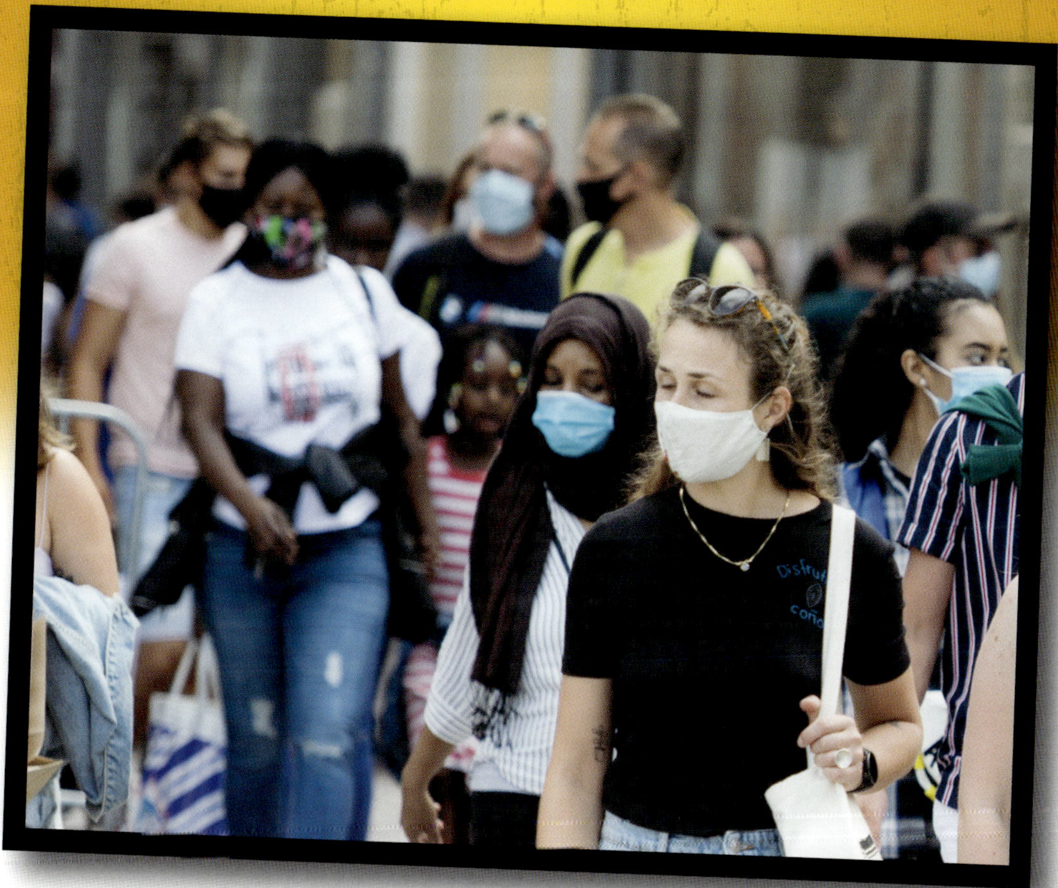

Millions of people caught the disease.

disease: an illness

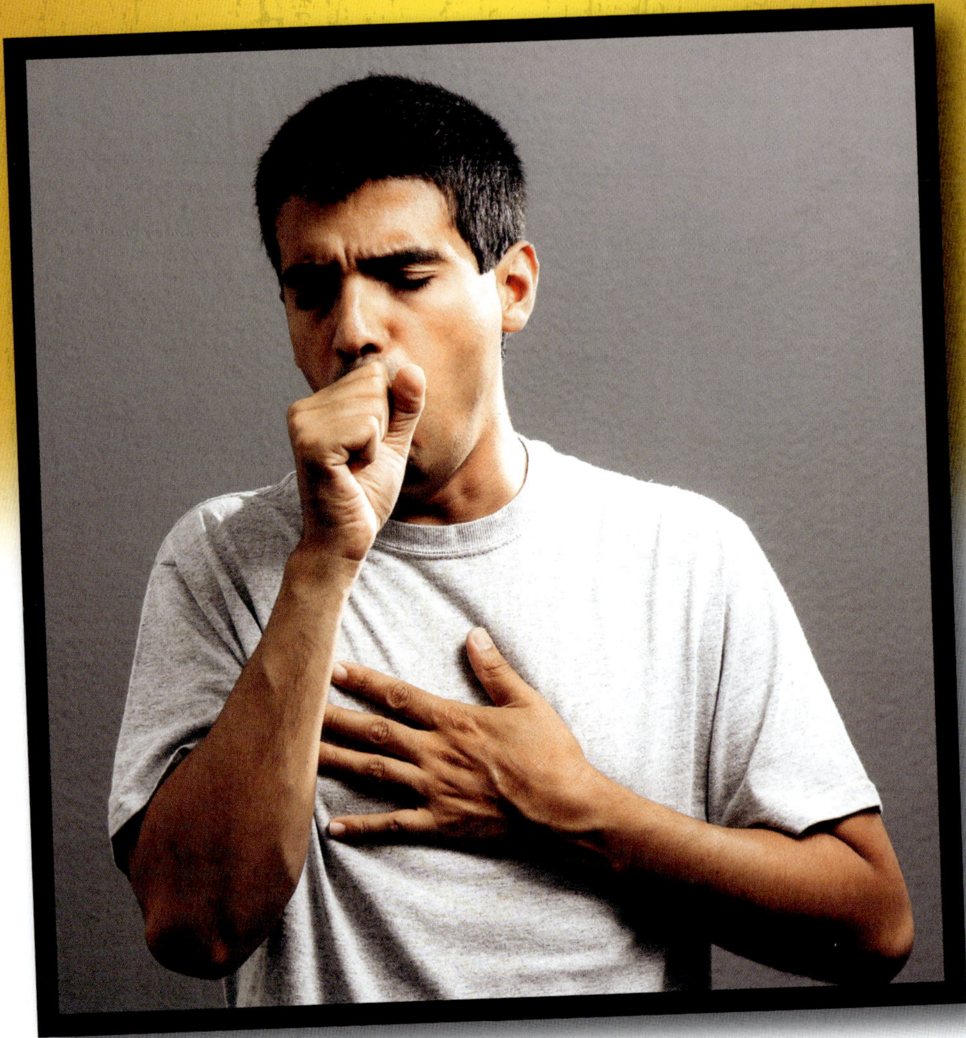

Some people with COVID-19 had fevers, coughs, and body aches. Others didn't feel sick.

Scientists think COVID-19 started in China.

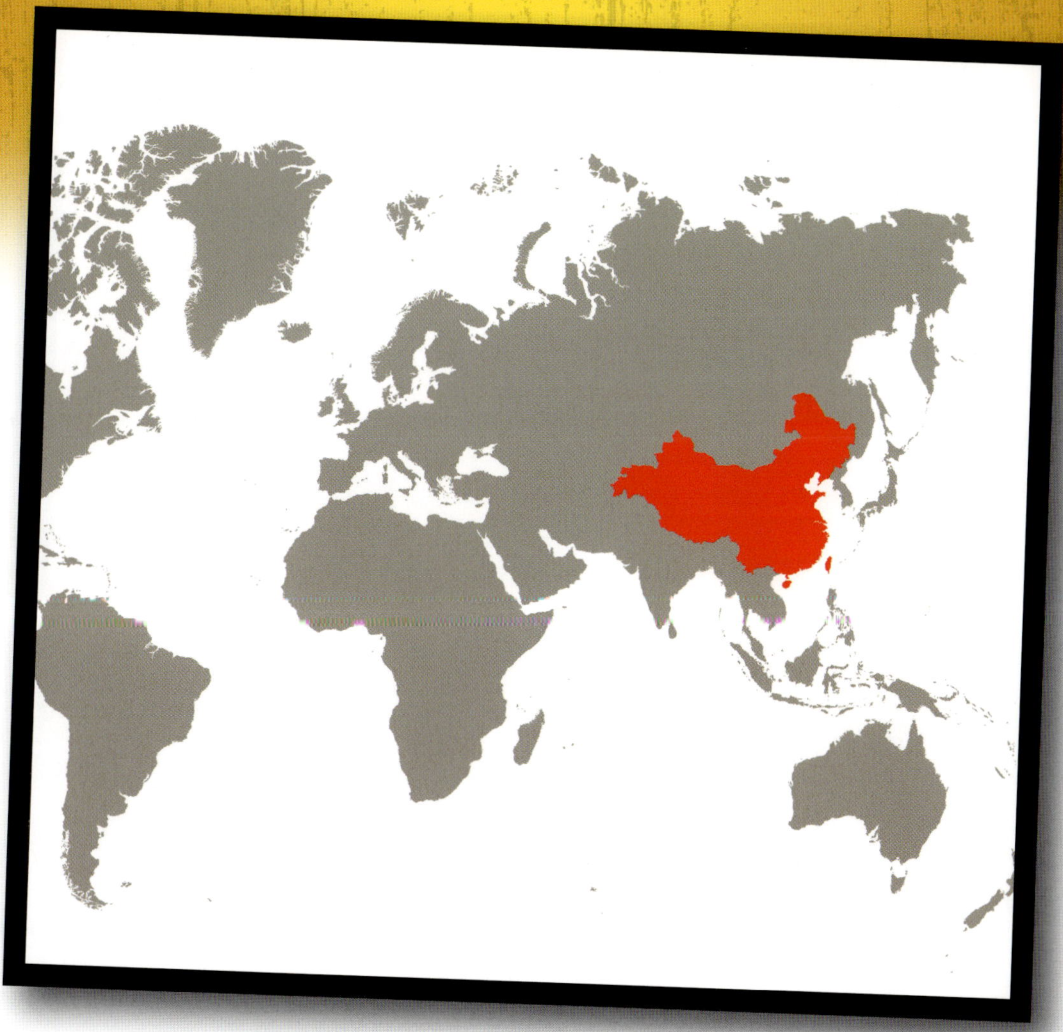

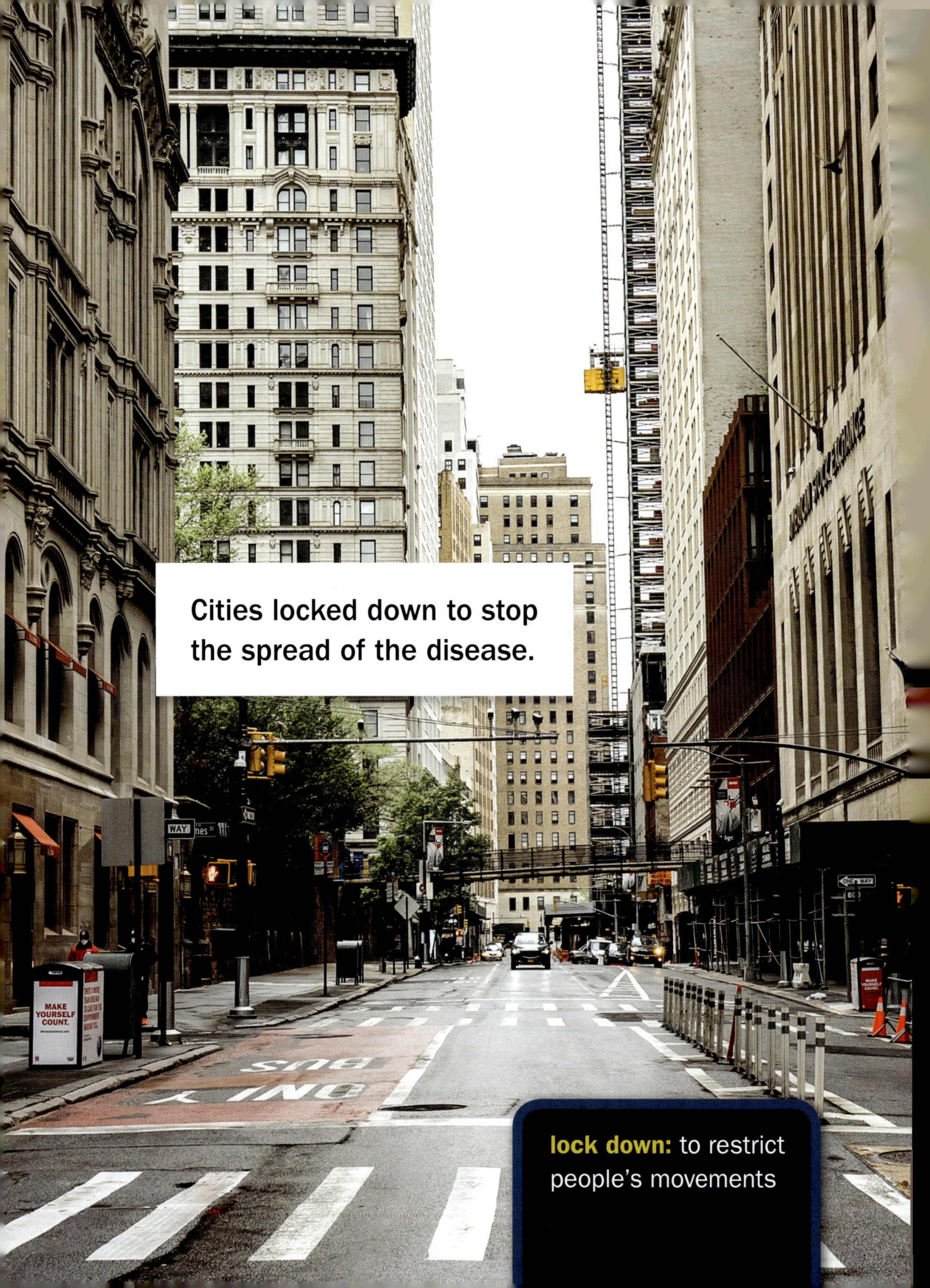

Cities locked down to stop the spread of the disease.

lock down: to restrict people's movements

But some people traveled and spread COVID-19 around the world.

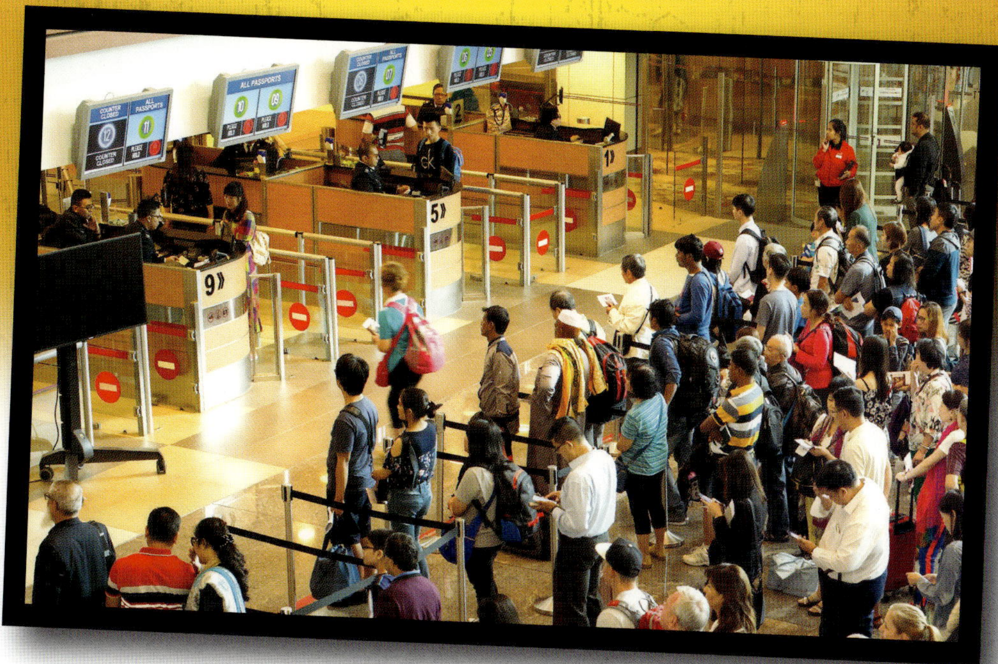

UP NEXT!

Coronaviruses and COVID-19.

What Causes COVID-19?

COVID-19 is caused by the SARS-CoV-2 virus.

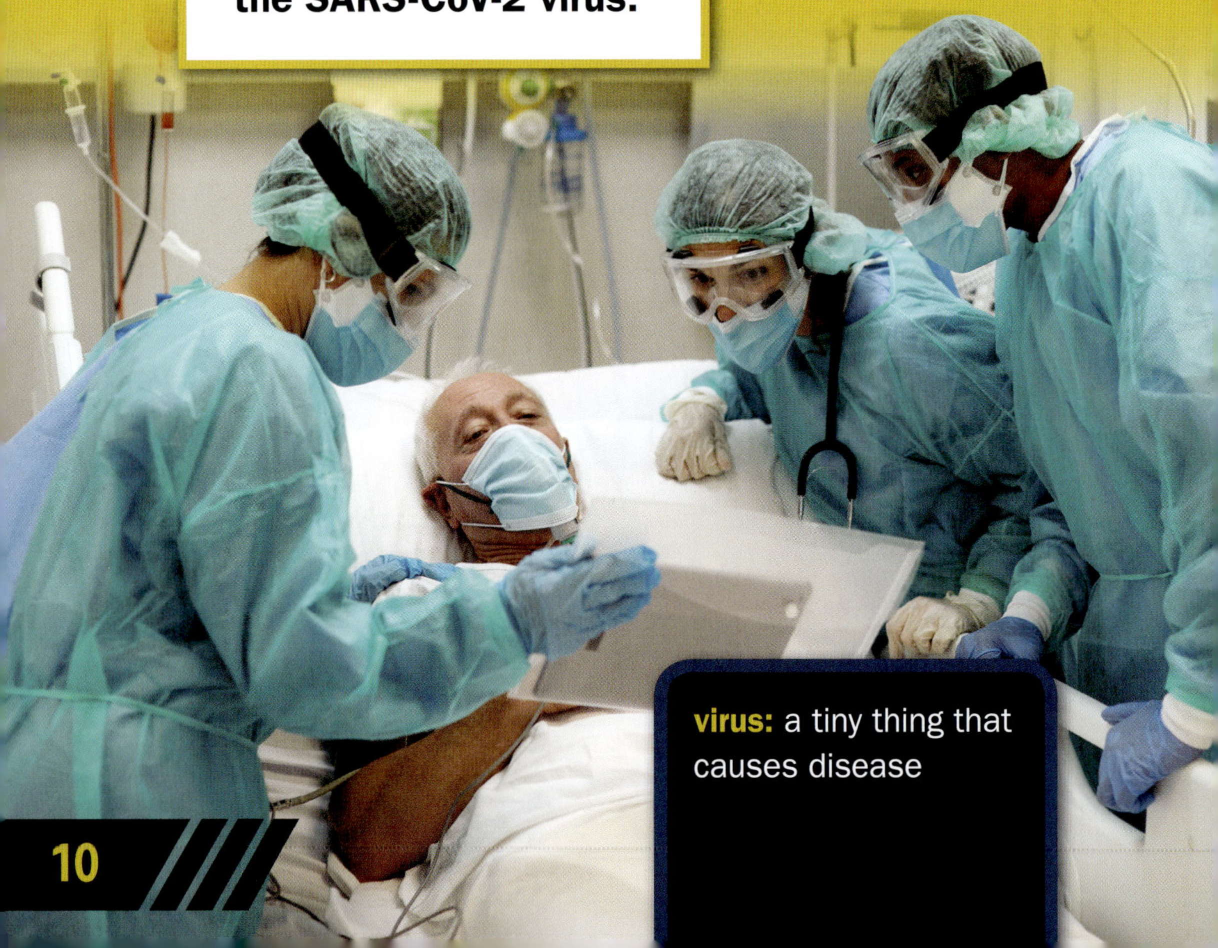

virus: a tiny thing that causes disease

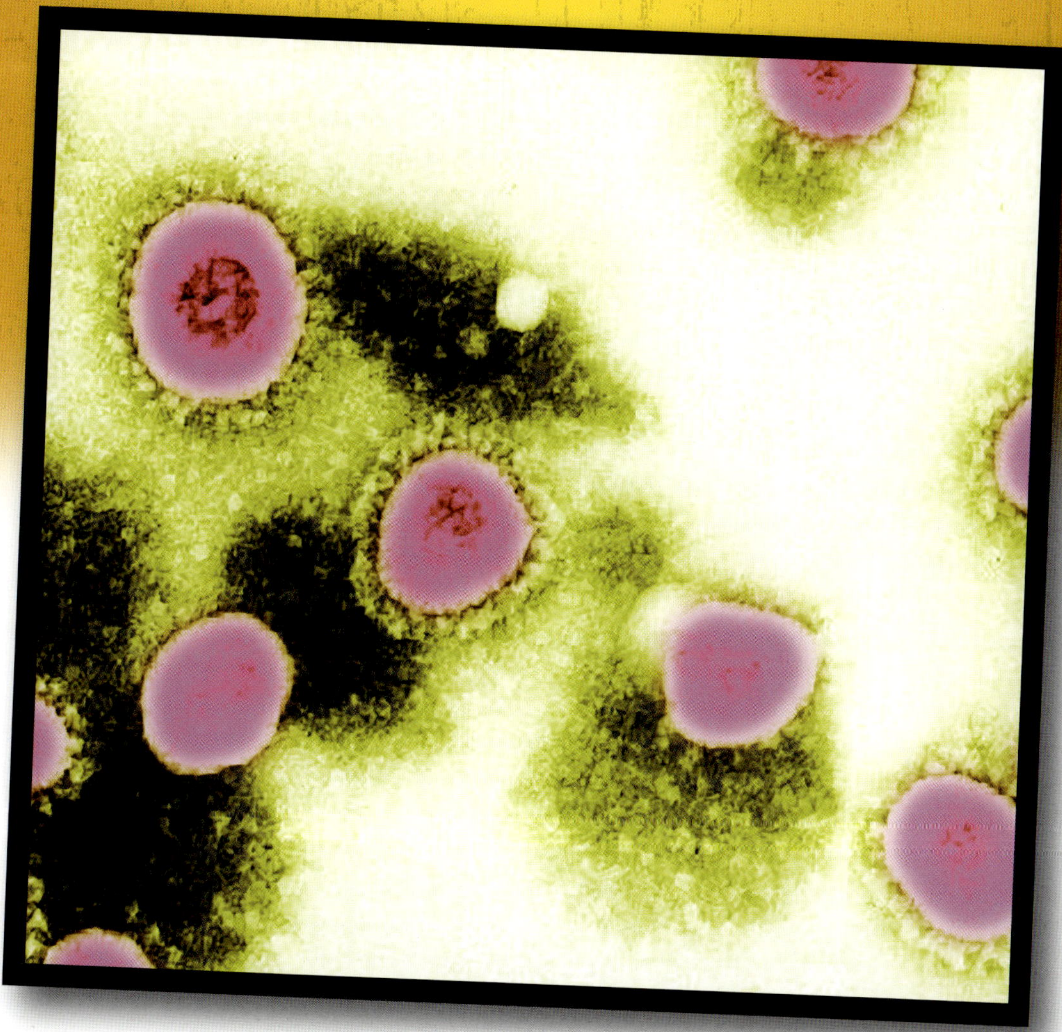

SARS-CoV-2 is a coronavirus. Coronaviruses cause different diseases.

UP CLOSE

The image on the right shows SARS-CoV-2.

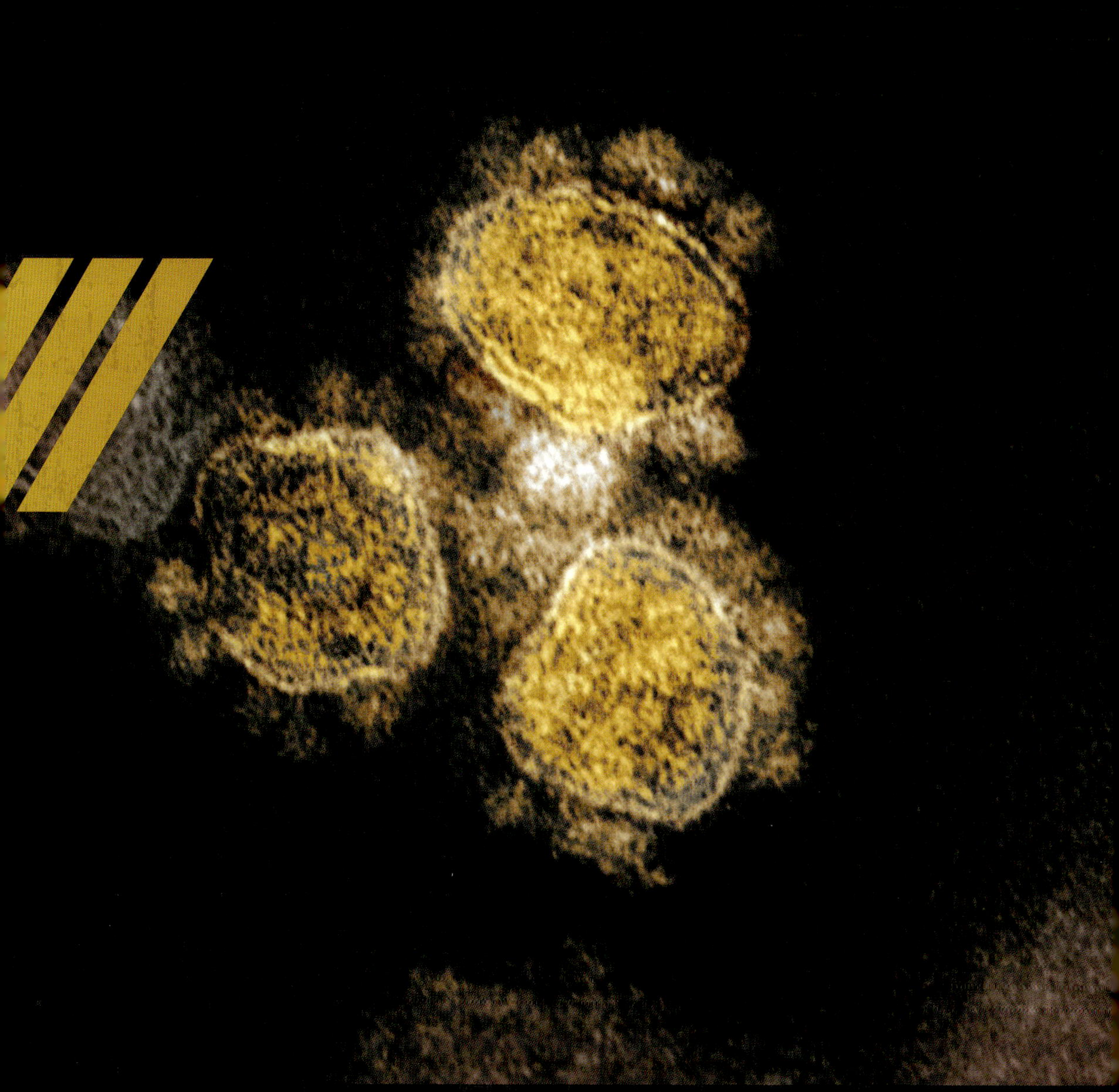

UP NEXT!

Fighting the virus.

Stopping the Spread

COVID-19 mainly spreads from person to person through the air.

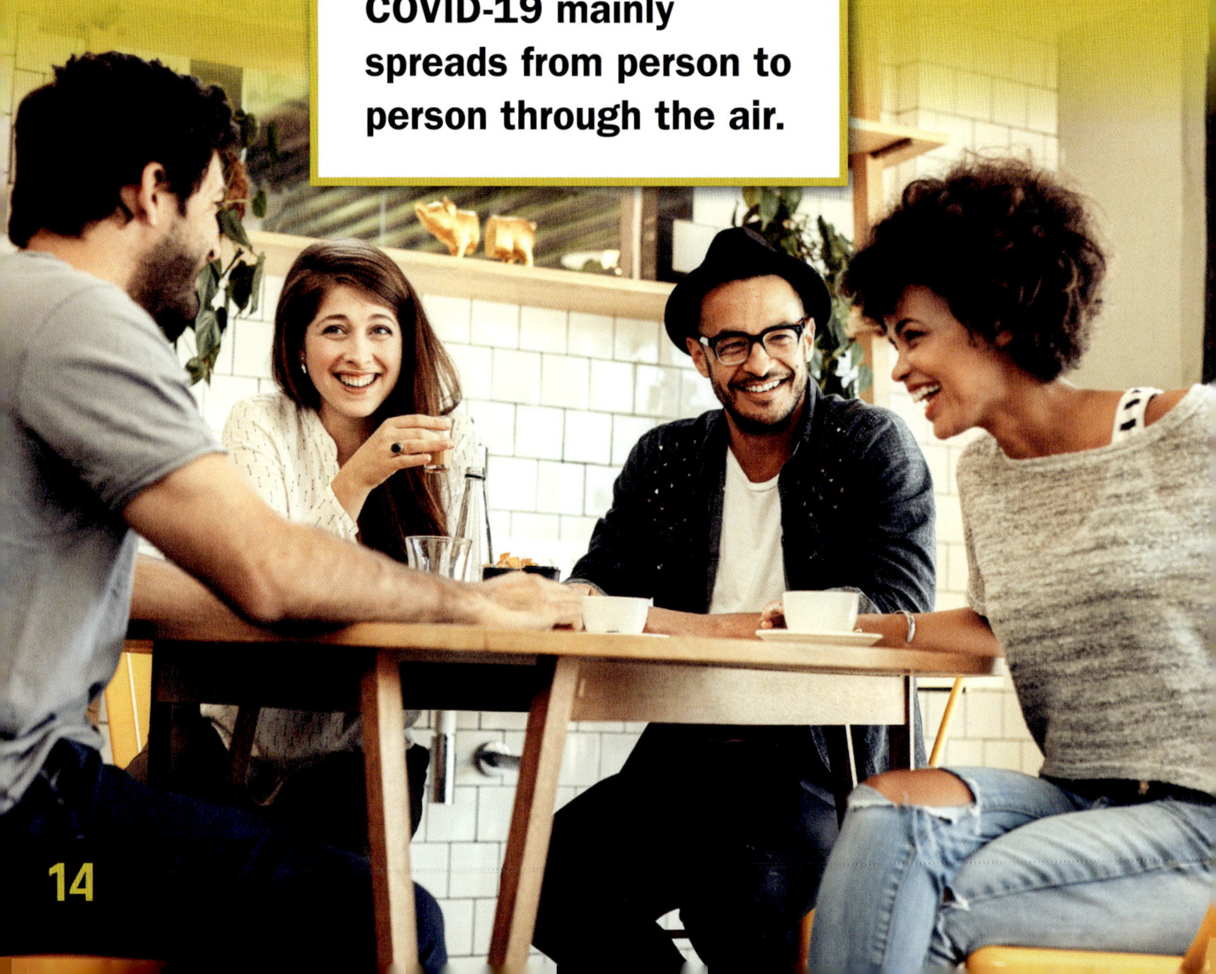

A cough or sneeze from someone with COVID-19 can spread the virus.

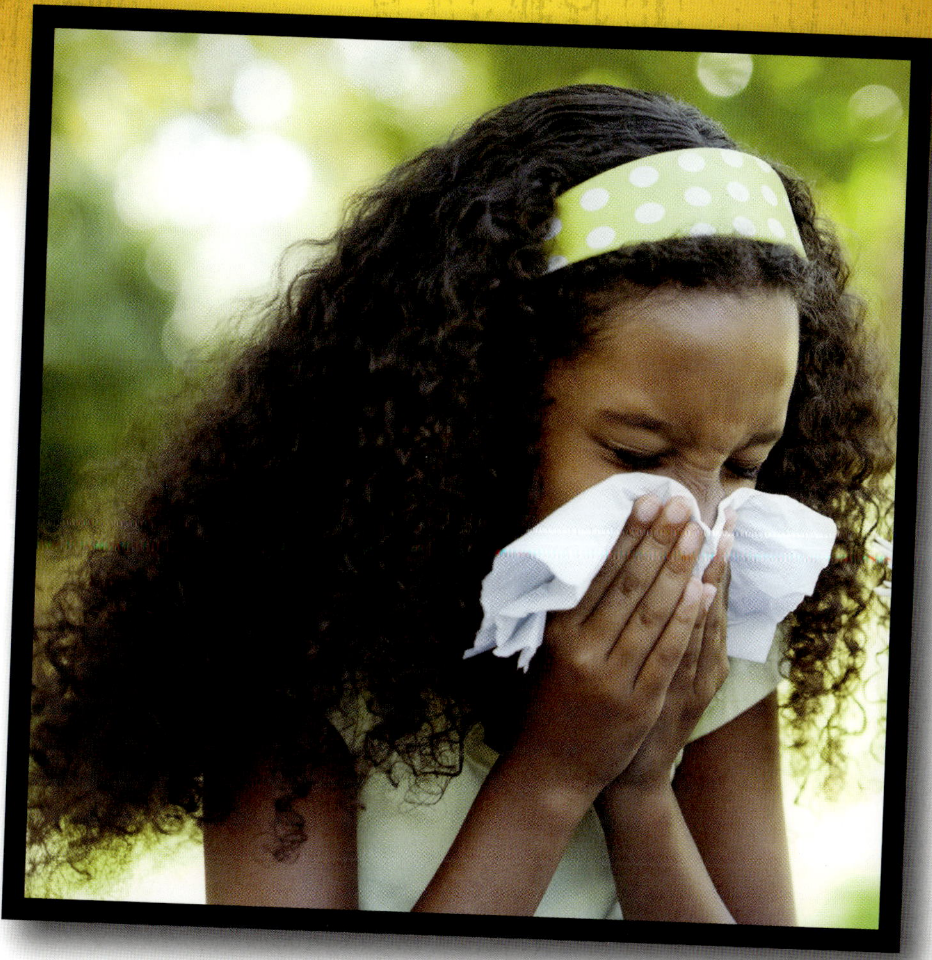

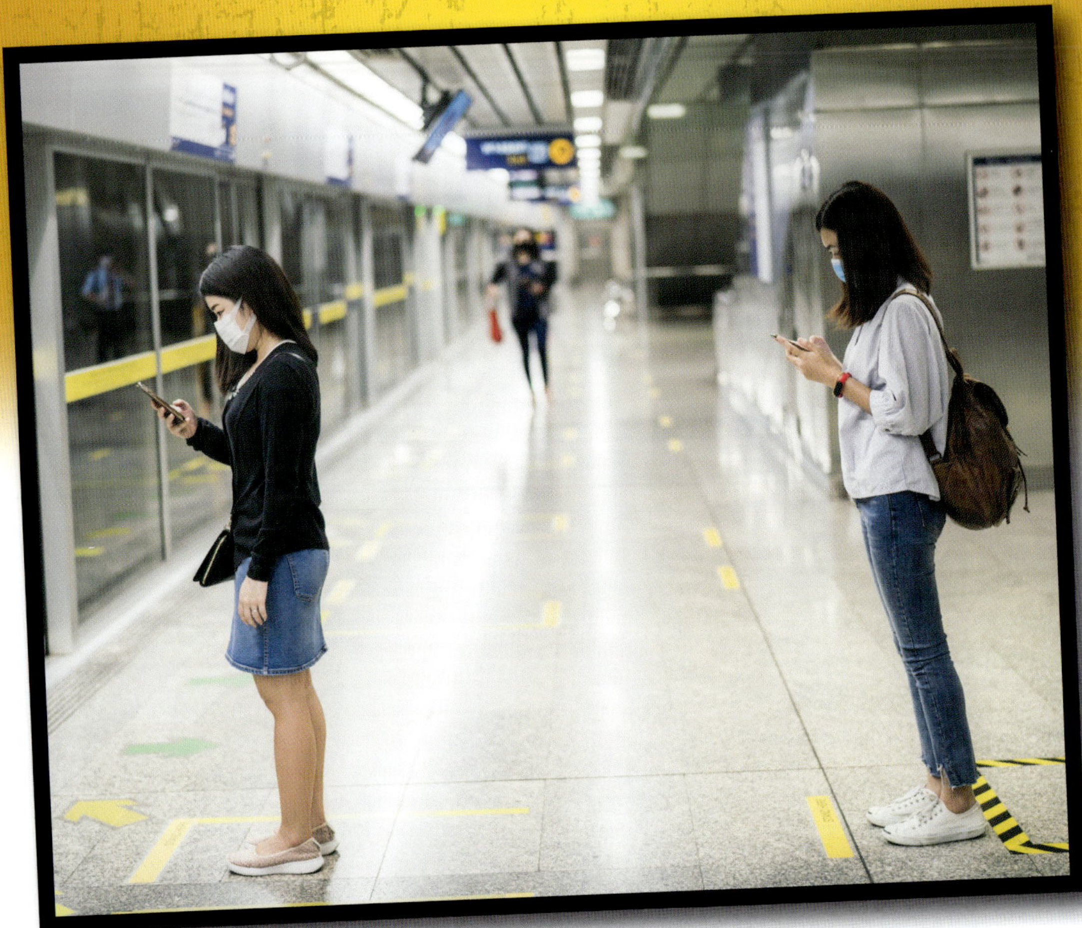

To stop COVID-19, many people stayed away from others.

Some worked and studied at home.

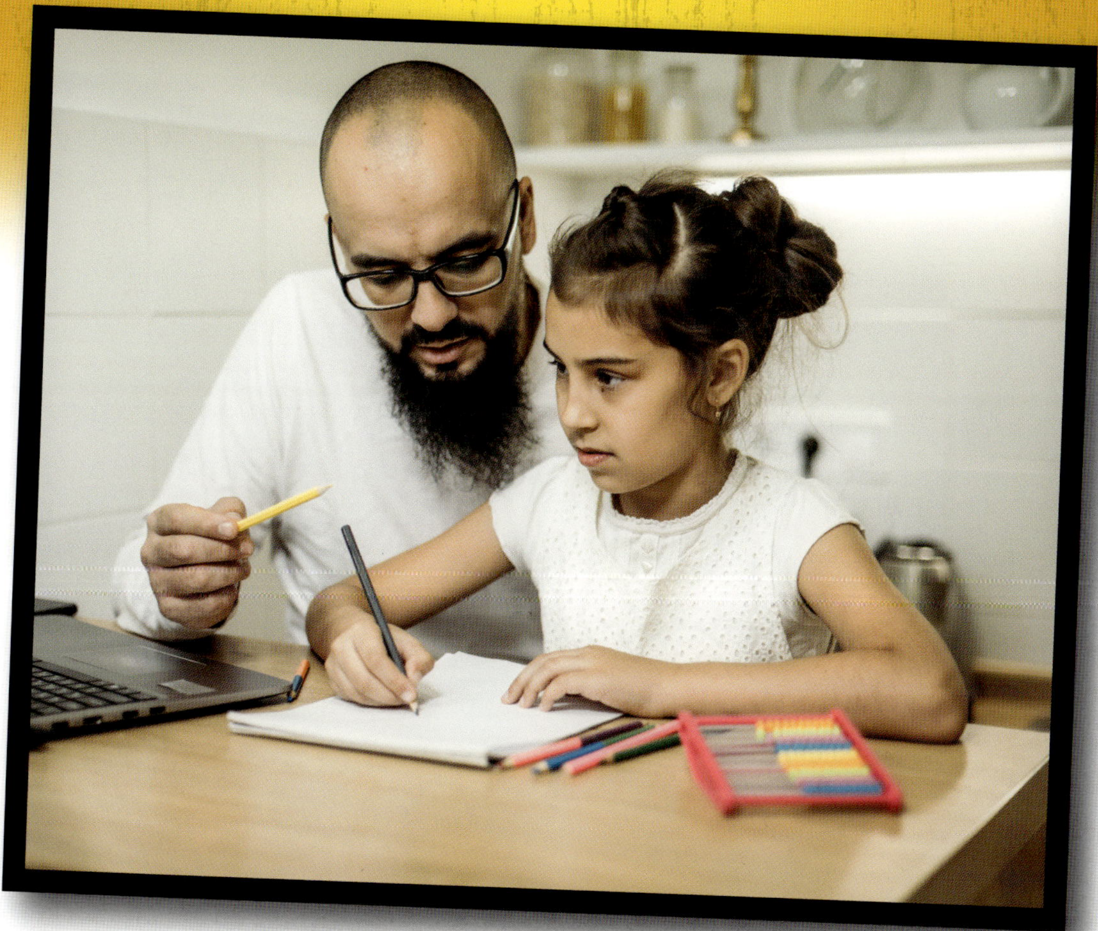

Many people talked to friends, family, and coworkers on computers.

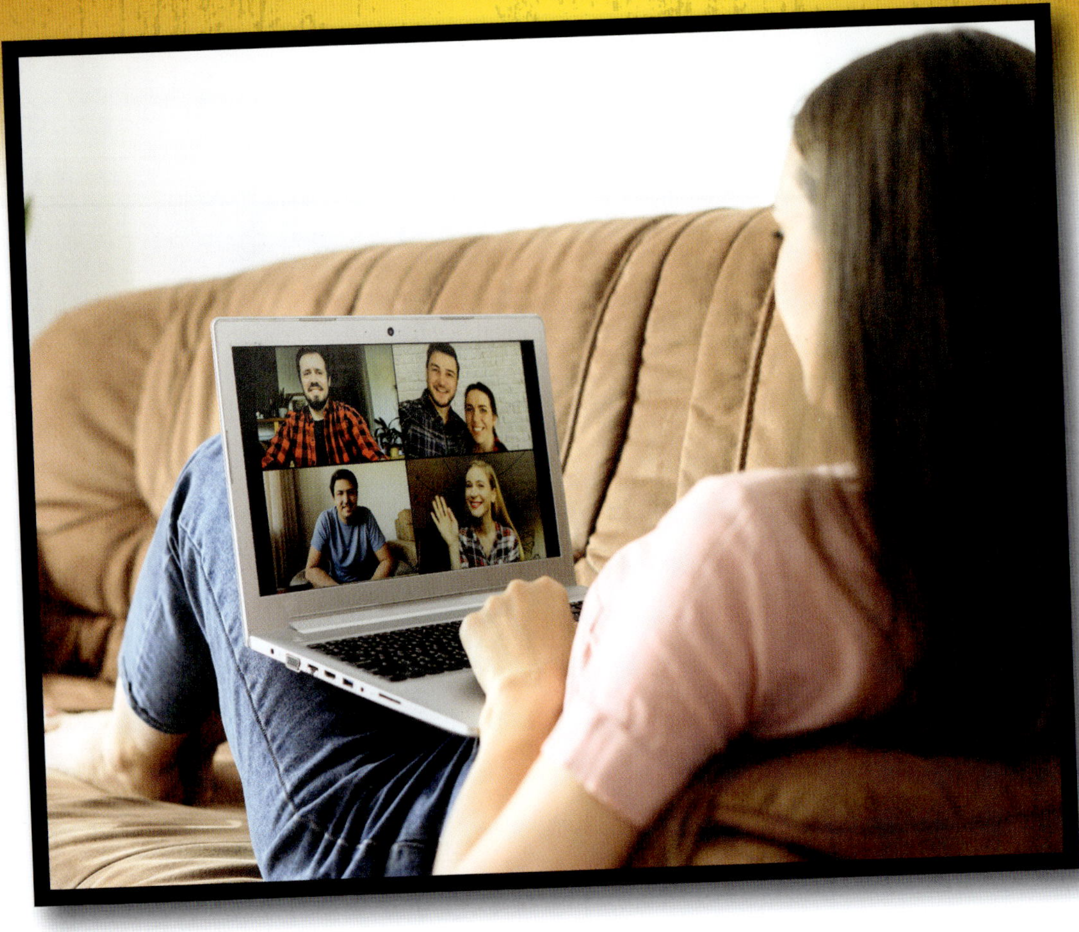

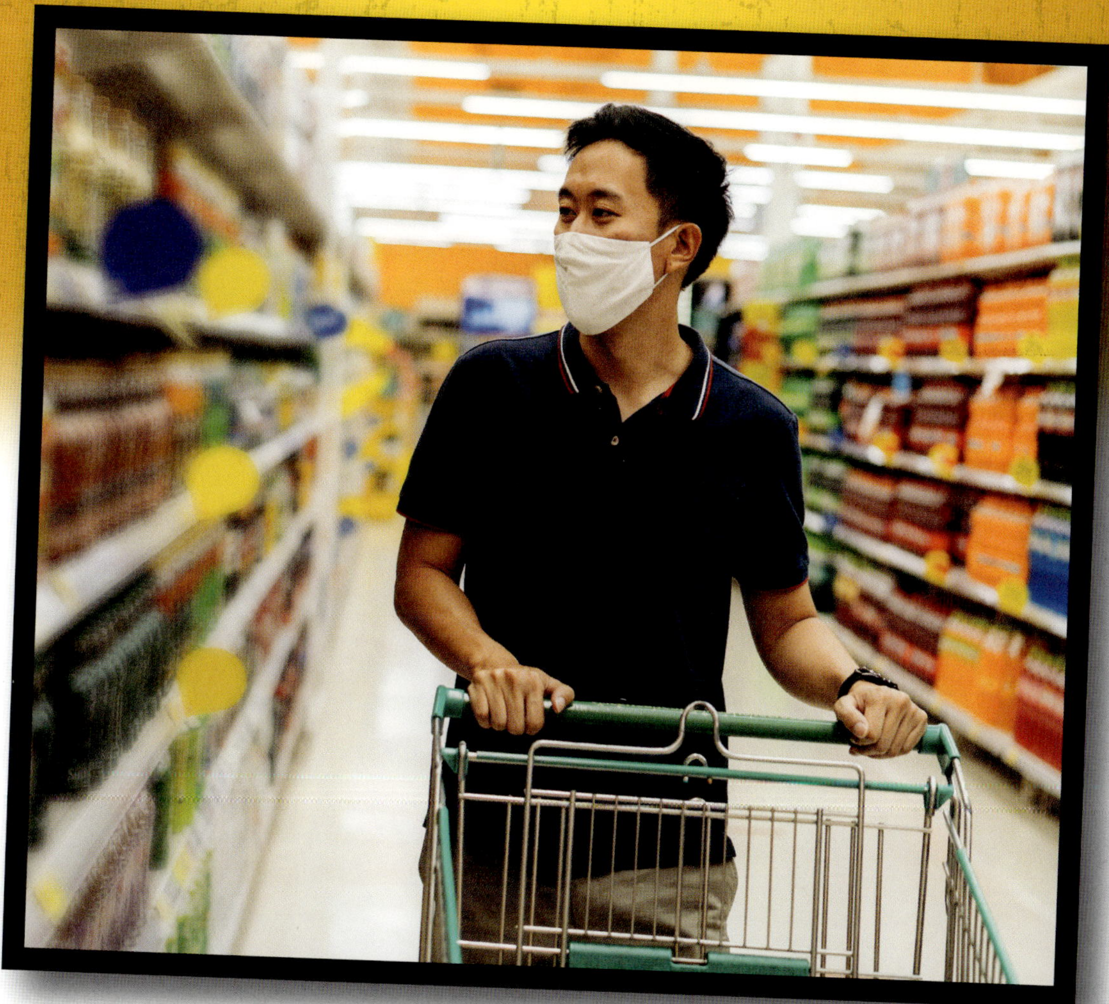

People wore masks in public places.

Many people worked together to stop COVID-19.

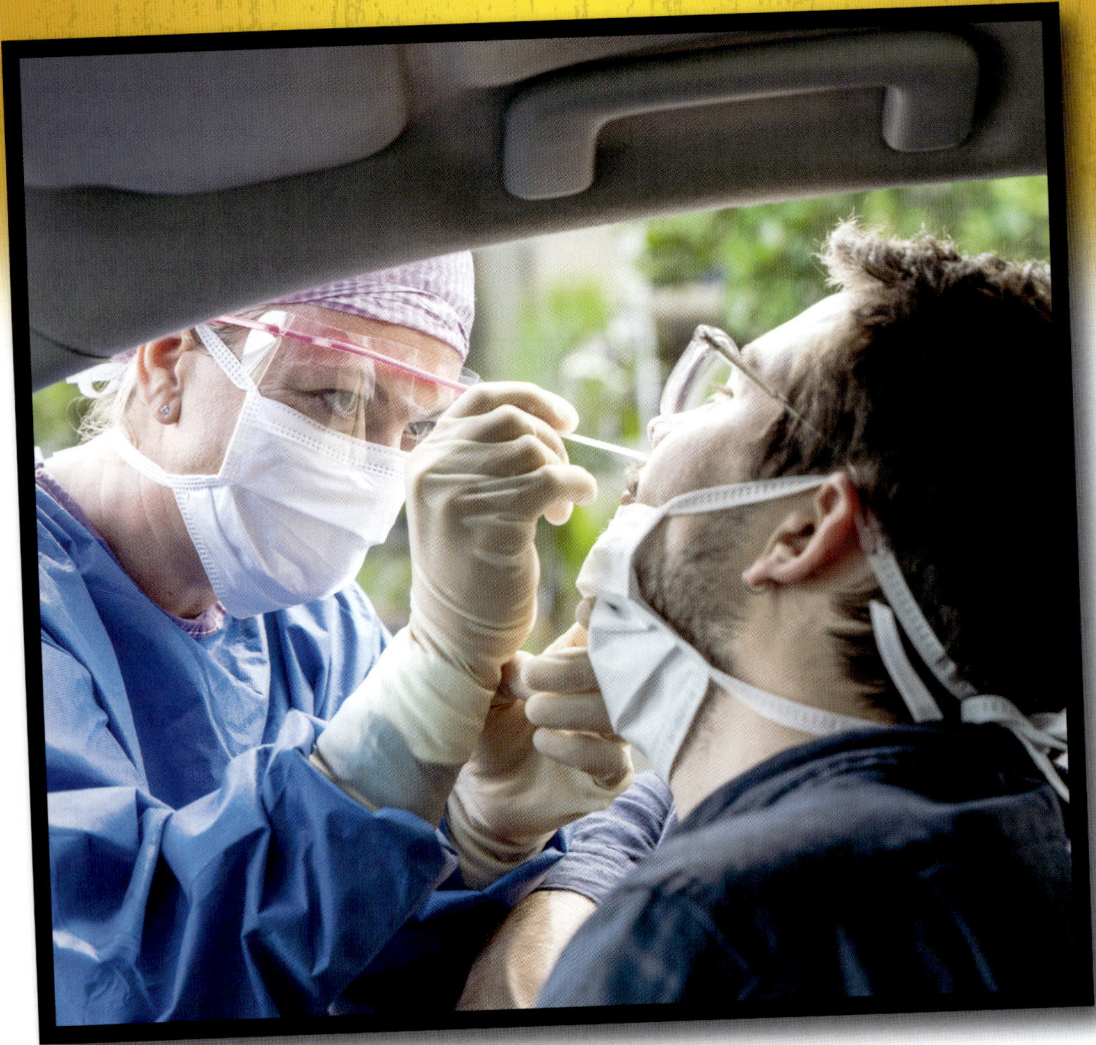

DOCTOR YOU!

Do you know which patient has COVID-19?

Patient A

sore throat
dry mouth
cough

Patient B

cough
body ache
fever

Answer: Patient B

Glossary

disease: an illness

lock down: to restrict people's movements

virus: a tiny thing that causes disease

Check It Out!

Coronavirus Facts for Kids
https://kids.kiddle.co/Coronavirus

Coronavirus: What Kids Can Do
https://kidshealth.org/en/kids/coronavirus-kids.html?ref=search

Facts about Coronavirus
https://kids.nationalgeographic.com/explore/science/facts-about-coronavirus/

Goldstein, Margaret J. *Understanding COVID-19*. Minneapolis: Lerner Publications, 2022.

Hudak, Heather C. *What Is a Virus?* New York: AV2, 2020.

Laughlin, Kara L. *What Is a Pandemic?* Mankato, MN: Child's World, 2020.

Index

Photo Acknowledgments

Image credits: David Benito/Shutterstock.com, p. 4; Elisabeth Aardema/Shutterstock.com, p. 5; Kleber Cordeiro/Shutterstock .com, p. 6; Omelchenko Andrii/iStock/Getty Images, p. 7; tetiana.photographer/Shutterstock.com, p. 8; joyfull/ Shutterstock.com, p. 9; Tempura/Getty Images, p. 10; Scott Camazine/Alamy Stock Photo, p. 11; NIAID-RML, pp 12–13; Jacob Lund/Shutterstock.com, p. 14; wavebreakmedia/ Shutterstock.com, p. 15; Travel man/Shutterstock.com, p. 16; Petryshak/Shutterstock.com, p. 17; Vadym Pastukh/ Shutterstock.com, p. 18; Twinsterphoto/Shutterstock.com, p. 19; zstock/Shutterstock.com, p. 20.

Cover: fpm/iStock/Getty Images.